Lígia Pelosi Mendonça
Ana Paula de L. Pfister
Arthur L. Mendonça

Respiratory muscle strength in individuals with OSAS

Lígia Pelosi Mendonça
Ana Paula de L. Pfister
Arthur L. Mendonça

Respiratory muscle strength in individuals with OSAS

And the relationship with the use of benzodiazepines

ScienciaScripts

Cover image: www.ingimage.com

This book is a translation from the original published under ISBN 978-3-330-76918-2.

Publisher:
Sciencia Scripts
is a trademark of
Dodo Books Indian Ocean Ltd. and OmniScriptum S.R.L publishing group

120 High Road, East Finchley, London, N2 9ED, United Kingdom
Str. Armeneasca 28/1, office 1, Chisinau MD-2012, Republic of Moldova, Europe
Managing Directors: Ieva Konstantinova, Victoria Ursu
info@omniscriptum.com

Printed at: see last page
ISBN: 978-620-8-62311-1

SUMMARY

SUMMARY

Obstructive sleep apnea syndrome (OSAS) is defined as the interruption of airflow for more than 10 seconds for an individual who has five or more episodes every hour of sleep during the night. It is the most serious occurrence of upper airway obstructive disorders which, in addition to disrupting sleep, can cause anxiety, irritability, insulin resistance, increase the risk of accidents and the development of cardiovascular diseases, contributing to a reduction in quality of life. Among patients with OSAS, it is common to use benzodiazepine drugs, which have been shown to induce sleep and reduce muscle tone. However, this study aimed to assess respiratory muscle strength in individuals with OSAS, as well as its relationship with benzodiazepines. Eighteen patients with the syndrome aged between 35 and 65 years were recruited from the offices of dentists specializing in sleep disorders in Formiga - MG and from a Postgraduate School in Sleep Dentistry in Belo Horizonte-MG. The volunteers filled in an identification questionnaire, their body mass index (BMI) was calculated, they answered the Mini-Mental State Examination (MMSE) and the IPAQ questionnaire. Finally, respiratory muscle strength (Pimàx and Pemàx) was measured. When the values obtained for Pimàx and Pemàx were compared with the predicted values, there was significance (p= 0.000), but when the difference in Pimàx and Pemàx was compared between patients who use the drug and those who don't, there was no statistical difference, with p=0.174 and p=0.537, respectively. It can be concluded that, in the sample analyzed, both inspiratory and expiratory muscle strength are reduced in patients with OSAS. When comparing the loss of strength in individuals taking benzodiazepine medication with those who did not, it was observed that there was no difference between the groups.

Keywords: Respiratory muscle strength. Obstructive sleep apnea syndrome (OSAS). Benzodiazepines.

1 INTRODUCTION

Obstructive sleep apnea syndrome (OSAS) is defined as the interruption of airflow for more than 10 seconds for an individual who has five or more episodes of apnea during seven hours of sleep in one night. These events can be perceived, analyzed and quantified by the test considered the gold standard in sleep disorders, polysomnography. It is a disease characterized by a collapse of the upper airways (UA) with a recurrent decrease in the calibre of the tubes, which can be complete or incomplete closure. It also presents repetitive episodes of hypoxia, hypercapnia and frequent awakenings (TARANTINO, 2008; PHAM AND SCHWARTZ, 2015).

There are different causes for the syndrome, but among them are some changes in the anatomy of the head and neck such as narrowing of the lateral pharyngeal walls, reduced activity of the pharyngeal dilator muscles in the elderly and also obesity, which is an important factor in the development of apnea and the only reversible one (AYAPPA and RAPOPORT, 2003; KUSHIDA et al., 1997; SHIMURA et al., 2005).

According to Roux et al. (2000), the syndrome is present in 9% of middle-aged men (between 30 and 60 years old), and in 4% of women in the same age group. Young et al. (2003) also state that there is a higher frequency of OSAS in the male population, in a ratio of 2:1.

The sleep of an individual with apnea is easy to identify by family members or roommates, as it is common to observe interruptions in breathing, snoring, moaning during exhalation and restlessness. The sufferer themselves may also notice symptoms such as headache, sore throat and dry mouth on waking, and nocturia (SILVA et al., 2009).

According to Marin et al. (2005) OSAS is the most serious occurrence of upper airway obstructive disorders, and is therefore capable of causing various alterations in the functioning of the body that go beyond sleep fragmentation, such as increased anxiety and irritability, indisposition, memory loss, increased risk of accidents and the chance of developing hypertension, insulin resistance and the risk of developing cardiovascular diseases, thus contributing to a reduction in quality of life. However, Peker et al. (2002) state that if the patient seeks appropriate treatment, it is possible to reduce or even prevent the onset of associated pathologies such as cardiovascular disorders.

Among patients with OSAS, there are those who use benzodiazepine medication. According to Rang et al. (2001), these drugs have a proven sleep-inducing and muscle tone-reducing action and are frequently used by these patients, as they also have an influence on reducing the anxiety and irritability often reported by apneics.

However, according to Katzung (2007), what is said about their real action on sleep disorders is more theoretical than practical, and little is known about the clinical impact of the effects of these drugs on individuals with OSAS. This is why we are interested in analyzing the influence of these drugs on the worsening of respiratory muscle strength in these patients, in order to see if there is a greater loss in those who use these drugs.

However, in view of the damage caused by OSAS and the small number of studies dedicated to observing the effects of this syndrome on respiratory functions, this study is justified.

The aim of this study was to assess respiratory muscle strength in individuals with Obstructive Sleep Apnea Syndrome (OSAS) and its relationship with the use of benzodiazepines, as well as evaluating Pimàx and Pemàx by comparing the values obtained with those predicted for age and gender according to the recommendations of Black and Hyatt in 1969, in addition to comparing whether individuals who use benzodiazepines have a greater deficit in Pimàx and Pemàx than individuals who do not use them.

The study was carried out in the offices of two dentists specializing in sleep disorders in Formiga, Minas Gerais, and in a post-graduate school of sleep dentistry in Belo Horizonte,

Minas Gerais, with 18 individuals aged between 35 and 65 with a medical diagnosis of OSAS. Initially, the patient answered an identification form (APPENDIX 02) which included personal data and other data such as BMI, existing pathologies, whether or not they smoked, and medication used. Cognitive status was then assessed using the Mini Mental State Examination (MMSE - APPENDIX 01). To check whether they were physically active, the International Physical Activity Questionnaire (IPAQ) (APPENDIX 02) was applied and the MVD 3000 Digital Manometer was used to measure respiratory muscle strength.

2. LITERATURE REVIEW

2.1 Respiratory system

2.1.1 Anatomy of the respiratory system

The respiratory system is made up of the nose, pharynx, larynx, trachea, bronchi and lungs and, depending on how it works, is divided into two parts: the conductive part and the respiratory part. The former is made up of the nose, pharynx, larynx, trachea, bronchi and bronchioles, tube-shaped structures whose function is to conduct air; the latter is made up of respiratory bronchioles, alveolar ducts, alveolar sacs and alveoli, which have a gas exchange function (TORTORA, 2000).

Air enters through the nostrils into the vestibule of the nose. The floor of its cavity is made up of bone tissue (hard palate) and muscle tissue (soft palate), the palate being responsible for dividing the nasal cavity from the oral cavity. The pharynx is a structure made up of muscles lined with mucosa and divided into the nasopharynx, buccopharynx and laryngopharynx. The larynx is made up of nine cartilages and the trachea continues up to the sixth thoracic vertebra. Also made up of cartilaginous rings, the trachea is divided into the right and left main bronchi. The right main bronchus is more aligned with the trachea, while the left main bronchus has a more acute and longer branching angle. Each main bronchus is further divided into smaller structures, the lobar bronchi and then segmental bronchi until they form the bronchioles which are further divided into terminal and respiratory bronchioles which are subdivided into alveolar ducts, alveolar sacs and, finally, the pulmonary alveoli (IRWIM AND TECKLIN, 2003; SPENCE, 1991).

The two lungs are located in the thoracic cavity and are the main respiratory organs. They are cone-shaped, have an apex, a base that rests on the diaphragm muscle, a costal face and a medial face where the pulmonary hilum is located, where bronchi, vessels and nerves enter and exit. Each of the lungs is surrounded by a serous sac called the pleura, which is divided into two leaflets: the pulmonary pleura and the parietal pleura. There is a liquid between them that allows one to slide smoothly against the other during variations in lung volume (DANGELO E FATTINI, 2000).

2.1.2 Physiology of the respiratory system

There are two factors that cause the lung to expand and contract: the movement of the diaphragm muscle, which lengthens and shortens the thoracic cavity, and the movement of the ribs, which increases and decreases the anteroposterior diameter of the thorax, ensuring effective inhalation and exhalation (GUYTON, 2002).

Inspiration is an active process in which the diaphragm contracts, the abdominal contents are pushed down and the ribs are moved outwards and upwards. This process generates an increase in the space inside the chest, decreasing the pressure inside and bringing the air flow into the lungs. When there is an increase in respiratory rate and tidal volume, which usually occurs during more intense activities, the external intercostal muscles and accessory muscles can also be recruited to provoke a more vigorous inhalation (COSTANZO, 1999).

According to Aires (1999) and West (2002), expiration is generally passive during basal breathing. During this process, the elastic tissues of the lungs and thorax will be distended as a result of the contraction of the inspiratory muscles and, consequently, potential energy will be retained in these tissues and released together with the retraction of the previously distended tissues, promoting expiration. The lung and chest wall, therefore, are elastic structures that tend to return to their equilibrium positions after being expanded during inspiration. During exhalation, the most important muscles are the abdominals, which, when they contract, generate an increase in intra-abdominal pressure, pushing the diaphragm upwards.

According to its movements during inhalation and exhalation, it is possible to conclude that the lung is normally a distensible and compact structure, and lung compliance is defined as a change in volume per unit change in pressure, which is approximately 200ml/cmH2O (IRWIM AND TECKLIN, 2003).

2.2 Respiratory muscle strength

Muscle strength is the ability of a muscle or muscle group to develop tension and force resulting from maximum effort, both dynamically and statically in relation to the demands made on it (KISNER AND COLBY, 1998).

The performance of the respiratory muscles depends, like that of any other muscle, on their strength, endurance and resistance to fatigue, but in addition, what will help determine the pressures generated in the respiratory system are the elastic properties of the lungs and chest wall. Therefore, respiratory muscle strength is defined as the maximum and minimum pressure generated within the respiratory system at a certain lung volume (IRWIM AND TECKLIN, 2003).

Inspiratory muscle strength is determined by the maximum inspiratory pressure (Pimàx) and expiratory muscle strength is determined by the maximum expiratory pressure (Pemàx). An efficient method for assessing respiratory muscle strength is the manovacuometer, a device that measures positive (manometer) and negative (vacuum) pressures. In order to measure Pimàx, inspiration must begin after a deep expiration (at residual volume level) and in order to measure Pemàx, it is important that expiration begins after a deep inspiration (at total lung capacity level). This measurement should be carried out with the airway occluded to prevent air escaping, and there should only be the orifice of the mouthpiece that keeps the glottis open. Maximum effort is also required. Some diseases can cause changes in the contractile strength of the muscles responsible for ventilation and, depending on the severity of the loss, can lead to weakness, fatigue or muscle failure (AZEREDO, 2002).

2.3 Obstructive sleep apnea syndrome - etiology and epidemiology of OSAS

In 1976, Guilleminault apud Avelino (2002) defined apnea as the obstruction of airflow in the upper airways for more than 10 seconds, with 30 events of apnea during sleep being considered severe. OSAS is characterized by a collapse of the upper airways due to a recurrent decrease in the calibre of the tubes, which can be complete or incomplete closure. It is a progressive, chronic and disabling disease (REIMÂO E JOO, 2000; VALERA, DEMARCO E ANSELMO, 2004).

According to Peker, et al. (2002), this syndrome affects up to 24% of the adult population, most of whom are elderly and men, and is present in 9% of middle-aged men and 4% of women (ROUX, CICONELLI AND FALOPPA, 2000).

Sleep has the REM stage (rapid eye movement) and the NREM stage (non-rapid eye movement). In OSAS sufferers, ventilation is not regular in REM sleep, tidal volume and respiratory rate vary, there is a reduction in VAS muscle tone compared to NREM sleep and at times the awakening threshold may be high. Therefore, the period of greatest risk for these patients is REM sleep with more severe and long-lasting events. Apnea can also occur during NREM sleep, but this is occasional (AYAPPA and RAPOPORT, 2003).

There are several factors that can lead to the development of OSAS. Anatomical changes to the head and neck often determine the state of apnea. Micrognathia, which is a delay in mandibular development, leads to a retroposition of the mandible, which is related to the posterior positioning of the tongue. There are also people who have a small oral cavity with a high possibility of narrowing of the VAS. Authors agree that narrowing of the VAS is most commonly seen in the retropalatal oropharyngeal region. In normal individuals, the upper airways have a larger lateral diameter than the anteroposterior diameter, unlike OSAS patients who have an anteroposterior diameter larger than the lateral diameter, which justifies a narrowing in the retropalatal region. The lateral pharyngeal walls may be responsible for this event. In addition, during inhalation, negative intrathoracic pressure is passed on to the upper airways, causing a reduction in the cross-sectional area of the pharynx. It is the balance between the pressure inside the chest and the abduction force of the pharyngeal muscles that maintains the patency of the airways (AYAPPA and RAPOPORT, 2003; KUSHIDA et a.l, 1997).

According to Martin (1997), other factors contribute to the development of the syndrome. Some authors say that with increasing age, the caliber of the upper airways decreases in both genders. Shimura et al. (2005) also state that obesity also has an influence on the occurrence of the disease. Around 70% of sufferers are obese, which can be determined by the body mass index (BMI) with a cut-off point > 30 to be considered at risk of obstructive sleep apnea. As for neck circumference, the cut-off point is 40 cm to be considered a predisposition to the syndrome and the site for measurement is the crico-thyroid membrane. The high amount of fat or soft tissue in this area is said to be responsible for apnea in obese people (IP et al., 2000).

2.3.1 Diagnosis and treatment

OSAS presents signs and symptoms that form the clinical diagnosis such as snoring, pauses in breathing constantly during sleep, restlessness when sleeping, feeling of being suffocated when waking up, lack of attention, too much sleep during the day, sexual impotence, noises during sleep, headache when waking up, noises, among others (VALERA, DEMARCO AND ANSELMO, 2004).

Polysomnography is considered the gold standard in the diagnosis of respiratory disorders resulting from sleep and records the electroencephalogram, electrooculogram, chin electromyography, oronasal flow, thoracic-abdominal movements and pulse oximetry, which allows respiratory events to be detected. Treatment includes general and specific measures. Some guidelines are part of it and can be decisive for the patient's improvement, such as avoiding alcoholic drinks and sedative drugs, losing weight for those whose cause is obesity, and avoiding sleeping in a supine position. As for specific measures, there are devices that provide positive airway pressure (CPAP), intra-oral devices (IOA) and surgery. The first option normalizes oxyhemoglobin saturation and is indicated for moderate to severe stages.

OAs work by retropositioning the jaw and can be adjusted. They are used for mild cases and in more severe cases when patients cannot adapt to CPAP. There are several surgical procedures, but in adults there is controversy, as little efficacy has been observed in the treatment of OSAS (TARANTINO, 2008).

2.4 Benzodiazepines

The first benzodiazepine drug was synthesized by accident in 1961 and, in a short space of time, became the most widely prescribed drug. Its best known and most important effects are on the central nervous system and are summarized as: reducing anxiety, sedation and inducing sleep, reducing muscle tone and coordination, as well as having an anticonvulsant effect. When these drugs are administered in conjunction with apnea, two effects stand out: sedation and sleep induction and a decrease in muscle tone. Widely used by patients with OSAS, benzodiazepines reduce the time it takes for the individual to fall asleep and increase the total duration of sleep for those who sleep less than six hours a night, and there is a relationship between reduced anxiety and sedation during sleep in these patients (RANG et al., 2001).

Benzodiazepines can lead to a reduction in REM sleep (rapid eye movement), which is related to dreams, and SW sleep (slow waves), which corresponds to the deepest level of sleep, but what is said about the effects of these drugs on sleep are assertions without much practical basis, but rather theoretical (KATZUNG, 2007).

With regard to the second effect related to OSAS, decreased muscle tone, it can be said that benzodiazepines inhibit polysynaptic reflexes and internuncial transmission. They reduce tone by an action independent of their sedative effect. Muscle hypertonia is a characteristic noted in anxiety states which can lead to muscle pain and headaches, and can be an advantageous drug in the medical clinic (KATZUNG, 2007; RANG et al, 2001).

However, as benzodiazepine drugs have been proven to be effective in reducing the anxiety and irritability that is usually reported in OSAS, the administration of these drugs is common for these patients, but there is still a lack of information about their real action in sleep disorders (KATZUNG, 2007).

3. MATERIALS AND METHODS

3.1 Type of study

This is a quantitative cross-sectional observational study, carried out in the offices of two dentists specializing in sleep disorders in Formiga - MG and in a postgraduate school in Sleep Dentistry in Belo Horizonte-MG after approval by the Research Ethics Committee of the Centro Universitàrio de Formiga (ANNEX 4).

According to Pereira (1995), observational studies are reserved for investigating naturally occurring situations. The researcher does not intervene, making it different from experimental studies. One of the main objectives of an observational study is to describe the classification of a parameter in the population (descriptive study), which helps to formulate a hypothesis.

Reis, Ciconelli and Faloppa (2002) state that in cross-sectional studies, the researcher must determine all the parameters at once, without a follow-up period.

3.2 Target population

The target population was formed by convenience and consisted of 18 individuals aged between 35 and 65 who were recruited at the offices of two dentists specializing in sleep disorders in Formiga - MG and at a post-graduate school in Sleep Dentistry in Belo Horizonte-MG before being treated by the professionals.

3.2.1 Inclusion criteria

- Signature of the ICF (APPENDIX 01);
- Preserved cognitive state according to the MMSE evaluation (ANNEX 01)
- Have a medical diagnosis of OSAS;
- Have hemodynamic stability at the time of collection (BP measurement - identification form - APPENDIX 02).

3.2.2 Exclusion criteria

- Did not sign the ICF (APPENDIX 01);
- Individuals who were smokers or former smokers (identification form - APPENDIX 02);
- Individuals with a BMI above 30 kg/m$^{2;}$ (identification form - APPENDIX 02);
- Active individuals according to the IPAQ (ANNEX 02);
- People with other cardiorespiratory pathologies and neuromuscular diseases (identification form - APPENDIX 02).

3.3 Instruments

3.3.1 Identification sheet

Prepared by the author of this study in order to characterize the sample. It consists of items related to the identification of the individual (name, age, gender, address, telephone number), specific data (medication in use, associated diseases, smoking), recording of vital data at rest (blood pressure), recording of anthropometric data (weight, height and BMI calculation) and recording of measured Pimâx and Pemâx values.

3.3.2 Anthropometric data

To measure weight (P), a G,TECH® digital scale was used, measuring up to 200kg, with a 50g division, duly calibrated, and for height (A), a COGEX® tape measure with a 0.1cm accuracy scale measured the point marked on the wall by the height of the individual who stood barefoot and with their head aligned.

The BMI value was later verified by calculating mass in kilograms divided by height in square meters (BMI= Kg/m$^{2)}$. In 1998, the World Health Organization (WHO) defined the cut-off points for BMI as: underweight with a BMI below 18.5 Kg/m2, normal weight with a BMI between 18.5 and 24.9 Kg/m2, overweight with a BMI between 25 Kg/m2 and 29.9 Kg/m2 and obese with a BMI above 30 Kg/m2. It also divided the obesity index related to mortality risk into three grades: pre-obese (BMI 25 to 29.9 Kg/m2), grade I or moderate obesity (BMI 30 to 34.9 Kg/m2), grade II or severe obesity (BMI 35 to 39.9 Kg/m2) and grade III or morbid obesity (BMI over 40 Kg/m2).

3.3.3. Mini Mental State Examination (MMSE)

The MMSE (ANNEX 01) was validated in 1994 by Bertolucci, Brucki and Campacci, and adapted more recently by Brucki et al. in 2003.

This study used the translation of the MMSE proposed by Bertolucci et al. (1994). The test consists of questions grouped into seven sets, each of which considers specific cognitive functions: temporal orientation has a maximum score of 5 points, orientation to space and place also has a maximum score of 5 points, registration of 3 words is worth 3 points, calculation and attention are worth 5 points, recall of 3 previously spoken words is worth 3 points, language is worth 8 points and visual constructive ability has a maximum score of 5 points.

1 point. The MMSE score can vary from zero to a maximum of thirty points. It's a simple scale and easy to apply, taking just 5 to 10 minutes (ALMEIDA, 1998).

Its results range from zero to 30 points, and an individual with altered cognition is considered to have a score of 13 for illiterates, 18 for those with one to seven years of schooling and 26 for those with more than eight years of schooling (BERTOLLUCI, BRUCKI AND CAMPACCI, 1994).

3.3.4 Physical Activity Questionnaire (IPAQ):

The International Physical Activity Questionnaire (ANNEX 02) was validated in 2001 by Pardini et al. and there are short and long versions. In this study, the patient was interviewed and the short version of the questionnaire was used, which consists of eight open-ended questions aimed at estimating the time spent per week on various levels of physical activity (light walking and medium to vigorous effort) and physical inactivity (sitting). However, the duration (minutes/day) and frequency (days/week) described in the questionnaire were analyzed and the individuals submitted to this questionnaire are classified as sedentary, insufficiently active A, insufficiently active B and active (GUEDES, LOPES E GUEDES, 2005).

3.3.5 Digital manometer

The manovacuometer used in this study is a digital, portable, microprocessor-based device, model MVD300®, which has a measurement unit of one cmH20 and an operating limit of 300cmH2O, previously calibrated. Inspiratory and expiratory pressures are read and stored through individual ducts.

This instrument measures Pimàx and Pemàx. The maximum inspiratory pressure (Pimàx) defines the strength of the muscles responsible for inhalation and the maximum expiratory pressure (Pemâx) defines the strength of the expiratory muscles (AZEREDO, 2002).

A 1.0 mm diameter hole was used during the measurement, as according to Shepherd et al. (2006) this minimizes the pressure generated by the facial muscles, avoiding a force measurement above the real value.

3.4 Procedures:

The study began after approval from the UNIFOR/MG Research Ethics Committee, opinion number 01/2012 (ANNEX 04). In a previous conversation, the dental professionals were informed about the aim of the study and, when they agreed to carrying out the data collection, they provided the days and times when it would be possible to meet the patients. They were informed about what was being studied and invited to take part in the research.

After signing the Informed Consent Form (ICF - APPENDIX 01), data collection began. Initially, the individual answered the identification form (APPENDIX 02), reporting their personal details, blood pressure was assessed to check hemodynamic stability, and weight and height were measured to calculate BMI. Specific data was collected, such as whether they were or had ever been smokers, whether they had any other illnesses, and what medication they were taking. After this, the Mini Mental State Examination (MMSE - ANNEX 01) adapted for Brazil by Bertolucci et al. (1994) was used to assess cognitive status; and the physical activity questionnaire (IPAQ - ANNEX 02) was used to assess their level of activity.

Respiratory muscle strength (Pimâx and Pemâx) was measured using a previously calibrated manovacuometer. First, the individual was instructed on the assessment through verbal explanations and demonstrations. In a sitting position with the torso and feet supported, the nasal orifices were occluded with a clip to prevent air escaping, and a mouthpiece was placed in the oral cavity to keep the glottis open during the passage of air, as shown in figure 1. To measure Pimâx, the patient exhaled deeply at the level residual volume and then inhaled with the mouthpiece in the oral cavity while being given standardized verbal stimuli by the researcher herself. To measure MEP, the patient had to take a deep breath at total lung capacity and then exhale with the mouthpiece in place so that all the stored air could come out, also listening to verbal commands. For the assessment of both Pimâx and Pemàx, three consecutive measurements were selected which did not exceed a difference of more than 5% or 10 points between them, with a maximum of five repetitions, and the highest value obtained between the three measurements was selected. An interval of one minute was given between each measurement.

The entire assessment procedure was carried out individually, by the same researcher and using the same equipment.

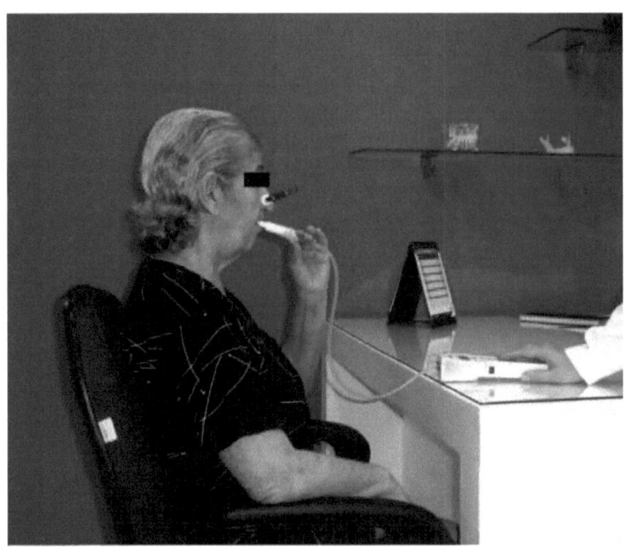

FIGURE 1- Measurement of Pimâx and Pemàx.

Source: Author's collection

3.5 Data analysis/processing:

Initially, a descriptive analysis was carried out on the data, which was presented in the form of percentages, means and standard deviations in graphs. The Kolmogorov/Smirnov test was then carried out to check the normality of the data, all of which was parametric.

To compare the values obtained for Pimàx and Pemàx with the values predicted for them and to compare whether individuals who use benzodiazepine drugs have a greater deficit in Pi màx and Pemàx than individuals who do not use them, the T-test was used.

The level of significance adopted for statistical treatment was 5% ($p < 0.05$).

The Mini Tab statistical package was used to prepare the database, as well as for the statistical analysis.

3.6 Ethical care:

This project was only carried out with the approval of the Internal Ethics Committee of the

Centro Universitàrio de Formiga - UNIFOR/MG (ANNEX 04). After this approval, data collection began. To this end, the research participants were informed that their identity and all their rights would be protected. Explanations about the study were given to those who were able to take part. Those who agreed to take part in the study signed an informed consent form (APPENDIX 01).

4. RESULTS

The volunteers were recruited from the offices of dentists specializing in sleep disorders in Formiga-MG and from a post-graduate school in sleep dentistry in Belo Horizonte-MG. A total of 22 patients were assessed, three of whom were excluded for having a BMI over 30 kg/m^2 and one for being a smoker. Of the 18 patients selected for the study, eight were female and ten were male, as shown in Graph 1.

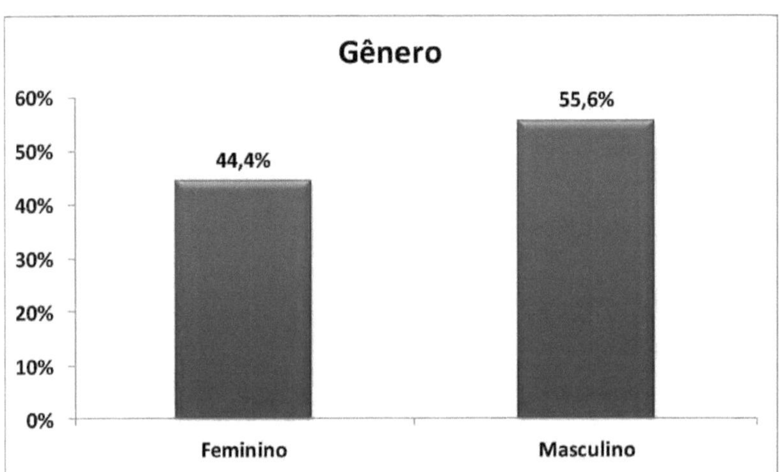

GRAPH 1- Distribution of genders in the population studied.

Source: by the author

Age ranged from 39 to 63 years, with a mean of 52.16 ± 7.19 years. Three individuals were aged between 35 and 45 (16.6%), eight between 46 and 55 (44.5%) and seven between 56 and 65 (38.9%).

Pimàx ranged from - 32 to - 78 cmH_2O with an average of - 57.33± 16.25 cmH_2O. Pemâx ranged from 43 to 179 cmH_2O with an average of 108.11± 36.14 cmH2O.

When comparing the Pimàx obtained with the Pimàx predicted for their ages and genders according to Black and Hyatt (1969), a statistical difference was observed (p=0.000), as shown in graph 2.

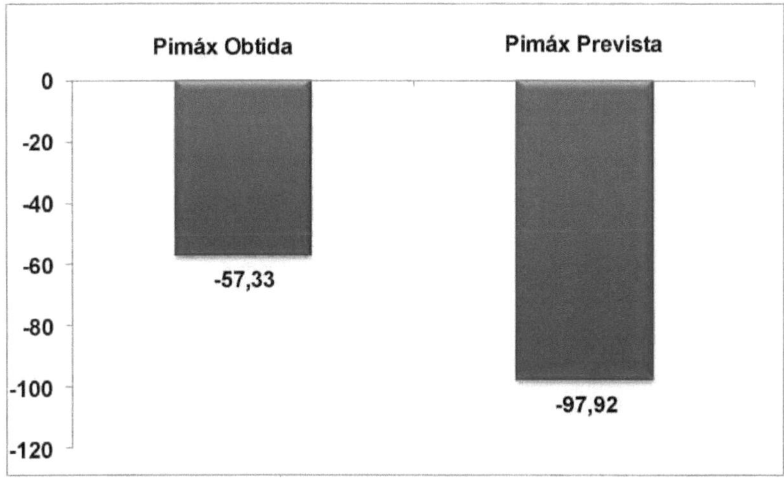

CHART 2 - Comparison of the mean Pimàx obtained with that predicted in cmH2O.

Source: by the author

When comparing the Pemàx obtained with the Pemàx predicted for their ages and genders according to Black; Hyatt (1969), a statistical difference was found (p=0.000), as shown in graph 3.

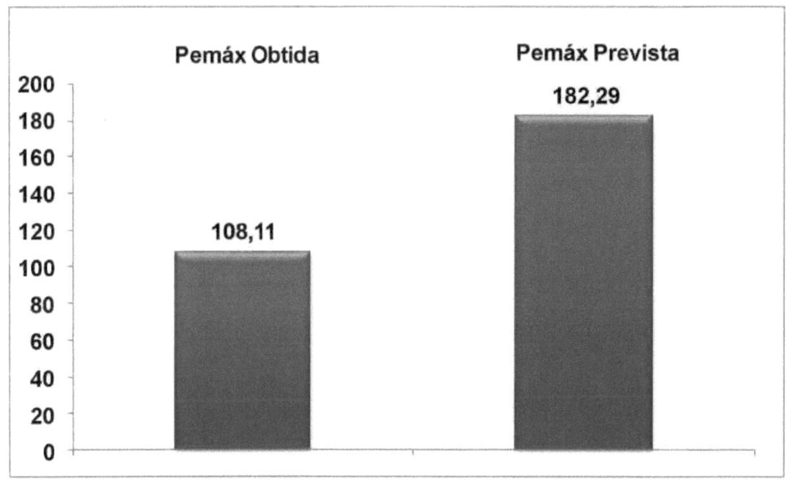

CHART 3 - Comparison of the mean Pemàx obtained with that predicted in cmH2O. Source: author

In order to analyze whether individuals who used benzodiazepine medication had a greater respiratory strength deficit than those who didn't, they were divided into two groups: the first with those who used medication, with 7 individuals (38.9%) and the second with those who didn't, with 11 individuals (61.1%). We calculated the predicted Pimàx minus the Pimàx obtained, comparing the means of the two groups. The same was done with Pemâx. The average values obtained are shown in Graph 4.

The comparison of the difference between the two groups' Pimàx showed p=0.174 and the comparison of the difference between the two groups' Pemâx showed p=0.537, which was not significant.

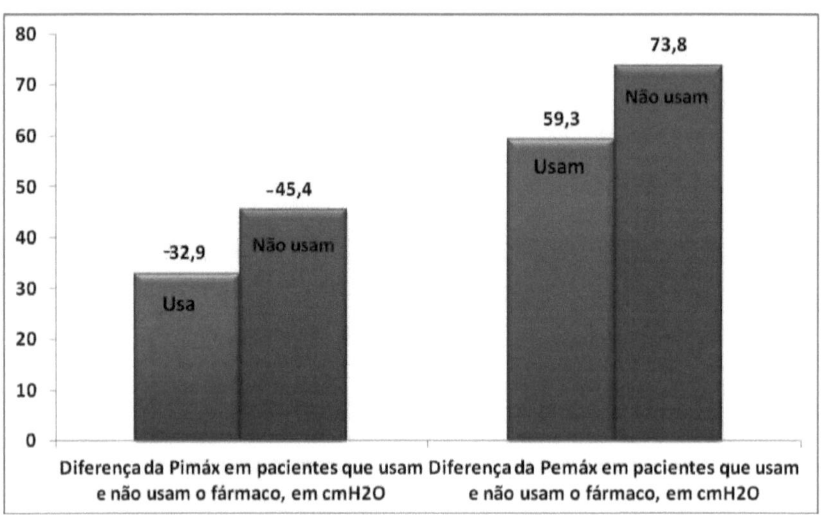

CHART 4 - Comparison of the means of the difference between the predicted Pimâx minus the obtained Pimâx and the difference between the predicted Pemàx minus the obtained Pemâx cmH2O.

Source: by the author

5. DISCUSSION

The aim of this study was to compare the respiratory muscle strength of 18 individuals with Obstructive Sleep Apnea Syndrome (OSAS) with the values predicted according to age and gender by Black and Hyatt (1969), using manovacuometry to measure Pimàx and Pemàx, as well as evaluating their relationship with the use of benzodiazepine medication. A predominance of men was observed, with 55.6% of the individuals.

According to Youg et al. (2003), there is a higher frequency of OSAS in the male population, in a ratio of 2:1. This is in agreement with the study by Dancey, et al. (2003) which evaluated 3,942 patients (2,753 men and 1,189 women) who underwent computerized polysomnography, and found that nocturnal apnea is significantly more frequent and more severe in men than in women. When analyzing the possible causes for this, it was observed that there was a statistical difference in the measurement of neck circumference, characterizing a greater volume in this region which predisposes to the syndrome; in addition to a higher BMI level among male patients, a risk factor for apnea. Ayappa and Rapoport (2003) also suggest that women have less resistance in their pharyngeal muscles.

In the study by Dahlqvist, et al. (2007) 801 patients with snoring underwent polysomnography (596 men and 205 women) in order to assess the following risk factors for nocturnal apnea: dimensions of the uvula and tonsils, velopharyngeal and lingual function, deviated nasal septum, mandibular position, neck circumference, weight and height, specific to each gender. It was found that in males, the factors that were related to an index of apnea events per hour of sleep >15 were: large tonsils, a high tongue and a wide orula. In women, large tonsils and mandibular retrognathism stood out as predisposing factors to a index> 15.

It is possible to observe that the factors that predispose individuals to the development of OSAS, as well as its aggravation, are varied, but there is general agreement that it is a prevalent occurrence in men, which corroborates this study and may justify the predominance of 55.6% in this population.

With regard to age, there was a range between 39 and 63 years, with an average of 52.16 ± 7.19 years, with the majority (44.5%) being between 46 and 55 years old, which is in line with Chien et al. (2010) who assessed 15 individuals aged between 40 and 65 years and obtained an average of 51.3 years.

According to the study by Sasai et al. (2011), which investigated changes in the breathing pattern of 30 OSAS sufferers, the average age was 35.8± 4.0 years, while Nunes (2008) found an average of 61.0± 8.6 years among 63 apneic and hypertensive volunteers.

Worsnop et al. (2000) aimed to determine whether some of the anatomical changes that predispose to Obstructive Sleep Apnea are age-dependent. In two groups of nine individuals, one aged between 20 and 25 years and the other between 42 and 67 years, it was found that there was a significant decrease in the activity of the intercostal muscles and, above all, the genioglossus and tensor palatini muscles, which help to keep the airway permeable, in the group of individuals aged between 42 and 67 years, justifying the greater chance of obstruction of the airways during sleep.

In this study, most of the patients reported working outside, having to deal with stressful events in their daily lives and some individuals mentioned having irregular sleep, waking up in the early hours of the morning or exchanging hours of nighttime sleep for daytime sleep. All these factors increase the risk of OSAS occurring or worsening, according to Ayappa and Rapoport (2003). Furthermore, the association of these factors with the changes resulting from ageing may justify the average age of 52.16 years found in this sample.

In the present study, when the Pimâx obtained was compared with the predicted Pimâx, there was a statistical difference ($p = 0.000$), showing a reduction in the inspiratory muscle strength of these patients, corroborating the study by Chien et al. (2010) which analyzed 15 men aged between 40 and 65 years with a recent diagnosis of severe OSAS compared with a control group. Muscle strength and resistance to fatigue of the diaphragm and vastus lateralis muscle were assessed by surface electromyography, as there was a hypothesis of peripheral skeletal muscle involvement. They concluded that the decrease in strength is significant in both the diaphragm and the vastus lateralis, but in relation to fatigue, there was significance only in the respiratory musculature, and it is justified that the inspiratory effort against partial or total occlusion of the VAS has a deleterious effect, causing muscle fatigue and consequent loss of strength.

However, in the study by Shepherd et al. (2006), 94 patients with a medical diagnosis of OSAS were analyzed, predominantly men (52 individuals) with a mean age of 47 years, and when evaluating Pimâx, it was found that there was no statistical difference between the value obtained and the value predicted according to the age and gender of the individuals. We also compared the Pimâx of patients with and without the syndrome, concluding that there was no difference either. The time of diagnosis and the severity of the patients investigated may be determining factors that justify the lack of significance found.

The decrease in inspiratory muscle strength observed in this study is possibly due to diaphragmatic fatigue caused by excessive repeated effort to overcome the occlusion of the upper airways, and also to the decrease in SatO2 often found in patients with OSAS, caused by intermittent hypoxia, as demonstrated by Sasai et al. (2011), who investigated changes in breathing patterns during one night's sleep in 30 patients with the syndrome. They were divided into moderate and severe OSAS groups, and one of their data points was the SatO2 assessment. They concluded that in the group of severe patients, those with the highest number of apnea events per hour, there was a significant decrease in SatO2, especially in the supine position, which has repercussions on oxygenation throughout the body, including the skeletal muscles.

In addition, the study by Nâcher et al. (2009) proved significance when it tested the hypothesis that intermittent hypoxia induces endothelial dysfunction of the diaphragm.

When comparing the Pemâx obtained with the Pemâx predicted according to their ages and genders according to Black; Hyatt (1969), a statistical difference was found (p=0.000), which is in line with the study by Lofaso et al. (2001) which analyzed the change in abdominal muscle activity with the inclusion of continuous positive airway pressure (CPAP). Before starting the protocol, it was found that six out of 12 patients were unable to sustain abdominal muscle contraction for a minimum period of time. Electromyography also showed that with the inclusion of nasal CPAP there was an increase in the activity of these muscles, leading to the conclusion that adequate oxygen supply is fundamental for good abdominal activity.

However, in the Su et al. study (2008), one of the objectives was to evaluate the Pemàx of individuals with OSAS before and after a night's sleep during polysomnography, analyzing 48 men. It was concluded that there was no correlation between Pemàx and the index of apnea events during sleep, in addition to an increase in expiratory muscle strength when comparing the values obtained with those predicted according to age and gender. The authors suggest that sleep has a restorative effect on the muscles responsible for breathing, regardless of the intensity of apneic impairment, and also that the respiratory muscles may be resistant to increased load and intermittent hypoxia during the night.

In the present study, the decrease in expiratory force is probably due to global hypoxia, which may be reducing oxygen supply to all skeletal muscles, including abdominal and peripheral muscles.

With regard to the loss of respiratory force in individuals taking benzodiazepines, it was found that there was no significant difference when compared to the loss in those who did not. Comparison of the difference between the Pimàx of the two groups showed p=0.174 and comparison of the difference between the Pemàx of the two groups showed p=0.537.

Hoijer et al. (1994) investigated 11 male patients with mild to moderate obstructive sleep apnea in a placebo-controlled, double-blind study. The influence of Nitrazepam on the frequency and severity of apneic events was analyzed, and it was concluded that the individuals who ingested the drug did not have a higher apnea index or changes in $SatO_2$. However, in this study, the drug was only administered for data collection, and the patients were not taking it continuously or for a long time. When it comes to analyzing loss of strength, you have to take into account a factor that is already in place and influential in the long term.

In the study by Nunes (2008), 63 apneic and hypertensive patients who used these drugs were divided into three groups and assessed for the rate of apnea events in relation to the use of the medication. It was observed that the magnitude of apnea was related in the group of patients taking a combination of antihypertensive and benzodiazepine drugs.

There is a scarcity of studies evaluating the loss of muscle strength related to the use of this drug, but in this study, the lack of a relationship between these two factors may be due to the fact that the amount ingested can be variable.

for each individual, as well as other factors that influence the occurrence of apnea, such as the anatomy of the head and neck (KUSHIDA et al., 1997), narrowing of the lateral pharyngeal walls, reduced activity of the pharyngeal dilator muscles in the elderly, , among others (AYAPPA and RAPOPORT, 2003).

Nerfeldt et al. (2004) carried out a study to assess the prevalence of benzodiazepine and alcohol abuse among OSAS sufferers, analyzing 96 individuals in Sweden. As far as the drug is concerned, no greater abuse was observed among the population with the syndrome.

This study had some possible limitations. Firstly, it was not possible to assess the date of onset of OSAS in each individual, as it is a nocturnal event that patients are often only able to identify when the disease has a detrimental effect on their daily lives. The index of apnea events per hour of sleep that determines the severity of OSAS was also not verified, which may have caused variability in the population studied, but all of them sought medical and dental help because they had daytime complaints that limited their daily functions, which characterizes moderate to severe apnea. Finally, the quantity, frequency and time of medication use were not assessed, and further studies are suggested to verify the correlation between these variables and loss of respiratory muscle strength.

In view of the above, further studies are also suggested to determine the time of onset and progression of the disease, as well as its severity.

6. CONCLUSION

According to the results obtained in this study, it was possible to observe that, in the sample analyzed, respiratory muscle strength is reduced in patients with Obstructive Sleep Apnea Syndrome (OSAS), both in Pimâx and Pemâx. And, when comparing the loss of strength in individuals who use benzodiazepines with those who don't, it was observed that there is no difference between the groups.

In this context, the importance of including physiotherapy in the multidisciplinary treatment of this patient is emphasized, since by strengthening the respiratory muscles, it is possible to minimize complications or consequences resulting from the loss of strength in OSAS. Specific exercises, appropriate instruments, respiratory and lifestyle reeducation, and guidance are all possible interventions that can provide efficient respiratory mechanics for a better quality of life for individuals.

REFERENCES

AIRES, MARGARIDA DE MELLO. **Physiology.** 2 ed. Rio de Janeiro: Editora Guanabara Koogan S.A. 1999. Pg. 514-525

ALMEIDA, O. P. **Mini Mental State Examination and the diagnosis of dementia in Brazil.** Arq Neuropsiquiatr 1998;56(3-B):605-612

AZEREDO, C. A. C.; **Modern respiratory physiotherapy**. 4ed. Barueri, SP: Manole, 2002 pg 79-84.

AVELINO, M. A. G.; PEREIRA, F. C.; CARLINI, D.; MOREIRA, G. A.; FUJITA, R.;

WECKX, L.L.M. **Polysomnographic evaluation of obstructive sleep apnea syndrome in children, before and after adenotonsillectomy.** Rev Bras Otorrinolaringol. V.68, n.3, 308-311, May/June 2002

AYAPPA I, RAPOPORT D. M. **The upper airway in sleep: physiology of the pharynx**. Sleep Medicine Reviews. Vol 7, No. 1, pp 9±33, 2003.

BERTOLUCCI PH, BRUCKI SM, CAMPACCI SR, Juliano Y. **The mini-mental state examination in a general population: impact of schooling**. Arq Neuropsiquiatr. 1994;52:1-7

BLACK, L. F.; HYATT, R. E. **Maximal respiratory pressures: normal values and relationship to age and sex.** American Review of Respiratory Disease, 1969.

Volume 99.

BRUCKI S. M.; NITRINI R.; CARAMELI P.; BERTOLUCCI P. H.; IVAN H.;

OKAMOTO I. H. **Sugestoes para o Uso do Mini -Exame do Estado Mental no Brasil. [Suggestions for utilization of the mini -mental state examination in Brazil]**. Arq Neuropsiquiatr 2003;61(3-B):777-81.

CHIEN, M-Y; WU, Y-T.; LEE, P-L.; CHANG, Y-J; YANG, P-C. **Inspiratory muscle**

dysfunction in patients with severe obstructive sleep apnoea. Eur Respir J 2010; 35: 373-380

COSTANZO, L.S. **Fisiologia**. Rio de Janeiro: Guanabara Koogan, 1999. Pg 157158

DAHLGVIST, J; DAHLGVIST, A; MARKLUND, M; BERGGREN, D; STENLUND, H; FRANKLIN, K. **Physical findings in the upper airways related to obstructive sleep apnea in men and women**. Acta Oto-Laryngologica, 2007; 127: 623_630

DANCEY, DV; HANLY, PJ; SOONG, C; LEE, B; JR. JS; HOFFSTEI, V. **Gender differences in sleep apnea**. CHEST 2003; 123:1544-1550.

DÂNGELO, José Geraldo; FATTINI, Carlos Américo. **Basic anatomy of organ systems.** Sâo Paulo: Atheneu Publishing House, 2000. Pg. 114.

GUEDES, D.P.; LOPES, C.C.; GUEDES, J.E.R.P.; **Reproducibility and validity of the International Physical Activity Questionnaire in adolescents**. Ver. Bras Med Esporte _ Vol. 11, N° 2 - Mar/Apr, 2005

GYTON, A. C.; HALL, J.E. **Treatise on Medical Physiology.** 10 ed. Rio de Janeiro: Editora Guanabara Koogan S.A, 2002. Pg. 406-415

HOIJER, U.; HEDNER, J.; EJNELL, H.; GRUNSTEIN, R.; ODELBERG, E.; ELAM, M. **Nitrazepam in patients with sleep apnoea: a double-blind placebo-controlled study**. Eur Respir J. 1994, 7, 2011-2015.

IP, MS; LAM, KS; HO, C; TSANG, KW; LAM, W. **Serum leptin and vascular risk factors in obstructive sleep apnea**. Chest. 2000;118(3):580-6.

IRWIM, SCOT; TECKLIN, JAN STEOHEN. **Cardiopulmonary physiotherapy**. 2 ed. Barueri-Sao Paulo: Editora Manole Ltda, 2003

KATZUNG, B. G. **Basic and clinical pharmacology**. 10 ed. Sao Paulo: McGraw-Hill, 2007. Pg. 310-313, 318

KISNER, C.; COLBY, L. A. **Therapeutic exercises**: fundamentals and techniques. 3. ed. Sao Paulo: Manole, 1998

KUSHIDA CA, Efron B, Guilleminault C. **A predictive morphometric model for the obstructive sleep apnea syndrome**. Ann Intern Med. 1997;127(8 Pt 1):581-7.

LOSAFO, F; D'ORTHO, M.P; FODIL, R.; DELCLAUX, C.; HARF, , A.; LORINOA.M.

Abdominal Muscle Activity in Sleep Apnea During Continuous Positive Airway Pressure Titration. CHEST, August 2001, vol. 120 no. 2 390-396

MARIN JM, CARRIZO SJ, VICENTE E, AGUSTI AG. **Long-term cardiovascular outcomes in men with obstructive sleep apnoea-hypopnoea with or without treatment with continuous positive airway pressure: an observational study.** *Lancet.* 2005;365(9464):1046-53.

MARTIN SE, MATHUR R, MARSHALL I, DOUGLAS NJ. **The effect of age, sex, obesity and posture on upper airway size.** Eur Respir J. 1997;10(9):2087-90.

NACHER, M.; FARRÉ, R.; MONTSERRAT, J.M.; TORRES, M.; NAVAJAS, D.;

BULBENA, O.; SERRANO-MOLLAR, A. **Biological Consequences of oxygen desaturation and respiratory effort in an acute animal model of obstructive sleep apnea (OSA).** Sleep Med. 2009 Sep;10(8):892-7.

NERFELDT, P.; GRAF, P.; BORG, S.; FRIBERG, D. **Prevalence of high alcohol and aenzodiazepine consumption in Sleep Apnea patients studied with blood and urine tests**. Acta Otolaryngol 2004; 124: 1187/1190

NUNES, JOSÉ PEDRO. **Usage of Antihypertensive Drugs and Benzodiazepines to Estimate Apnea/Hypopnea Index in Arterial Hypertension**. Clinical and Experimental Hypertension, 30:143-150, 2008

WORLD HEALTH ORGANIZATION (OMS). **Obesity preventing and managing the global**

epidemic. Geneva: WHO, 1998 (Report of a WHO Consultation on Obesity).

PARDINI, R; MATSUDO, S.; ARAÙJO, T.; MATSUDO, V.; ANDRADE, E.;

BRAGGIO, G.; ANDRADE, D.; OLIVEIRA, L.,; FIGUEIRA, A.J; RASO, V. **Validation of the international physical activity questionnaire (IPAQ - version 6): pilot study in young Brazilian adults.** Rev. Bras. Ciên. e Mov. Brasilia v. 9 n. 3 p. July 2001

PEKER, Y., HEDNER J., NORUM, J., KRAICZI, H., CARLSON, J. **Increased Incidence of Cardiovascular Disease in Middle-aged Men with Obstructive Sleep Apnea: A 7-Year Follow-up**. Am J Respir Crit Care Med Vol 166. pp 159165, 2002

PEREIRA, Mauricio Gomes. **Epidemiology theory and practice**. Rio de Janeiro: Guanabara Koogan,1995

PHAM L. V.; SCHWARTZ A. R. The pathogenesis of obstructive sleep apnea. **J Thorac Dis.** 2015;7(8):1358-72.

RANG, H.P.; DALE, M.M.; RITTER, J.M.; FLOWER, R.J.; **Pharmacology**. Rio de Janeiro: Elsevier Editora Ldta., 2007. Pág. 537-539.

REIMAO R, JOO SH, **Mortality of obstructive sleep apnea**. Rev Assoc Med Bras. 2000 Jan-Mar; 46(1): 52-6

REIS, F. B.; CICONELLI, R. M.; FALOPPA, F. **Scientific research: the importance of methodology**. Rev Bras Ortop., Rio de Janeiro, v. 37, n. 3, mar. p. 51-55, 2002.

ROUX F, D'AMBROSIO C, MOHSENIN V. **Sleep-related breathing disorders and cardiovascular disease.** Am J Med 2000:108:396-400.

SASAI,T; INOUE,Y.; MATSUO,A.; MATSUURA,M.; MATSUSHIMA, E. **Changes in respiratory disorder parameters during the night in patients with obstructive sleep apnoea**. Respirology 2011; 16, 116-123.

SHEPHERD, K.L.; JENSEN, C.M.; MADDISON, K.J.; HILLMAN, D.R.; EASTWOOD, P.R.

Relationship Between Upper Airway and Inspiratory Pump Muscle Force in Obstructive Sleep Apnea. CHEST 2006; 130:1757-1764

SHIMURA R, TATSUMI K, NAKAMURA A, KASAHARA Y, TANABE N, TAKIGUCHI Y, et al. **Fat accumulation, leptin, and hypercapnia in obstructive sleep apnea- hypopnea syndrome.** Chest. 2005;127(2):543-9.

SILVA GA, SANDER HH, ECKELI AL, FERNANDES RMF, COELHO EB, NOBRE F. **Basic concepts on obstructive sleep apnea syndrome.** Rev Bras Hipertens vol.16(3):150-157, 2009.

SPENCE, Alexander P. **Basic human anatomy**. Sâo Paulo: Manole, 1991. Pág. 516 a 523.

SU, M-C; CHIN, C-H; CHEN, Y-C; HSIEH, Y-T; WANG, C-C; HUANG, Y-C; LIN, MC. **Diurnal Change of Respiratory Muscle Strength in Patients with Sleep- disordered Breathing**. Chang Gung Med J 2008; 31: 297-303

TARANTINO, A. B. **Doenças pulmonares.** 6 ed. Rio de Janeiro: Guanabara Koogan, 2008. Pag. 457-467

TORTORA, GERARD J. **Corpo humano: fundamentos de anatomia e fisiologia.** 4 ed. Porto Alegre: Artmed Editora, 2000. Pg. 407

VALERA FCP, DEMARCO RC, ANSELMO-LIMA WT. **Obstructive sleep apnea and hypopnea syndrome (sahos) in children**. Rev Bras Otorrinolaringol. 2004 Mar-Apr; 70(2): 232-7.

WEST, J.B. **Respiratory Physiology**. 6 ed. Barueri, SP: Manole, 2002. Pag. 89-91.

WORSNOP, C; KAY, A; KIM, Y; TRINDER, J; PIERCE, R. **Effect of age on sleep onset-related changes in respiratory pump and upper airway muscle function**. J Appl Physiol 88: 1831-1839, 2000.

YOUNG T, FINN L, AUSTIN D, PETERSON A. **Menopausal status and sleep-disordered**

breathing in the Wisconsin Sleep Cohort Study. Am J Respir Crit Care Med. 2003;167(9):1181-5.

APPENDIX

APPENDIX 01 - Informed Consent Form

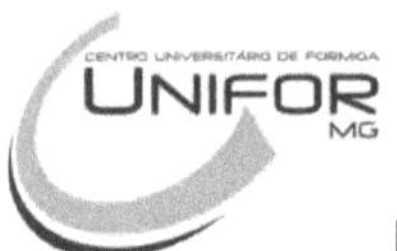

FORMIGA UNIVERSITY CENTER

Decree published on 05/08/2004

Sponsor: Fundaçâo Educacional Comunitària Formiguense - FUOM

INFORMED CONSENT FORM

Me, ,

nationality ______________________________ currently aged _________ years old

age, marital status, profession address

, ___________________________________RG , I am being invited to take part in a study called "Evaluation of respiratory muscle strength in patients with Obstructive Sleep Apnea Syndrome (OSAS) and the relationship with the use of benzodiazepines", whose objectives and justifications are: to define whether individuals with the syndrome have a reduction in diaphragm muscle strength and to assess whether those who use anxiolytic drugs (benzodiazepines) have greater impairment compared to those who do not. If the reduction in respiratory muscle strength and peak flow is proven, physiotherapeutic intervention is necessary in order to increase the strength of the respiratory muscles and prevent complications of the disease.

I will take part in the study by filling in an identification form which will include my details (name, age, address, telephone number, gender, medications I take, whether I am or have ever been a smoker, whether I have any other illnesses, and also blood pressure, weight and height measurements for later calculation of body mass index). I will then take the Mini-Mental State Examination, which will assess spatial orientation (ability to orient oneself in relation to objects, people and one's own body), memory, attention, verbal command and writing. To assess whether I do physical exercise and my level of activity, I will answer the IPAQ questionnaire and also perform a respiratory muscle strength test in which I will pull and blow air from my lungs into a device called a manovacuometer. I've been warned that I can expect, according to the results obtained by the research, benefits such as: guidance on the treatment best suited to my case and the values obtained by the tests I've taken. On the other hand, I have received the necessary clarifications about the study, bearing in mind that it is a research study and positive or negative results will only be obtained after it has been carried out, and that this study is free of any discomfort and possible risks of any kind that may occur during the course of the research.

I am aware that my privacy will be respected, i.e. my name or any other data or element that could in any way identify me will be kept confidential. I have also been informed that I can refuse to take part in the study or withdraw my consent at any time without having to give reasons, and that if I wish to leave the study, I will not suffer any damage to the assistance I have been receiving.

I am guaranteed assistance throughout the research, as well as free access to all additional information and clarifications about the study and its consequences, in short, everything I want to know before, during and after my participation.

However, having been advised of the content of all of the above, and having understood the nature and purpose of the aforementioned study, I hereby give my free consent to participate, being fully aware that there is no financial value to be received or paid for my participation, and being informed that I will not incur any expenses as a result of my participation in this research, so there will be no reimbursement.

The researchers involved in this project are Ana Paula de Lourdes Pfister, Ligia Pelosi Mendonça, linked to the Centro Universitàrio de Formiga - UNIFOR-MG in relation to this research and I can contact them by telephone at (37)91995859, (37) 9944 7441.

Ant, from ___ from ____________

Research subject

Name ____

Signature ____

Researcher responsible

Name ____

Signature ____

Researcher

Name ____

Signature ____

APPENDIX 02 - Identification Questionnaire

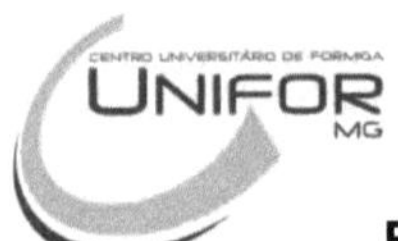

FORMIGA UNIVERSITY CENTER

Decree published on 05/08/2004

Sponsor: Fundaçâo Educacional Comunitària Formiguense - FUOM

Identification Questionnaire

1. IDENTIFICATION

Name ____

Address____

Age Phone number__

Gender ( ) M ( ) F

2. checking clinical stability

Arterial Pressure:/mmHg

3. ANTHROPOMETRIC DATA

Weight: _____Kg

Height: _____ m

BMI: Kg/m^2

4. SPECIFIC DATA

Are you or have you ever been a smoker? ( ) YES ( ) NO

Do you have another illness? ( ) YES ( ) NO What is it?

Medicines in use: ______________________________________

5. RESPIRATORY MUSCLE STRENGTH MEASUREMENTS

Pimàx:;; ;

Pemâx:;; ;

Source: by the author

ANNEX

ANNEX 01 - Mini Mental State Examination

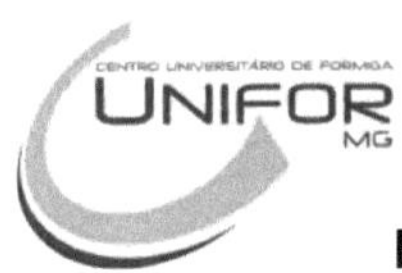

FORMIGA UNIVERSITY CENTER

Decree published on 05/08/2004

Sponsor: Fundaçâo Educacional Comunitària Formiguense - FUOM

MINI MENTAL

NAME ____

AGE DATE____________________

Cutting points

YEARS OF SCHOOLING: illiterate 13

1 to 7 years _______________ 18

8 or more years _____________ 26

Maximum score	Patient score	
5		**Temporal orientation:** day , month ______ , year ____ , day of the week ____ , hours_ _(0 a 5)
5		**Spatial orientation:** Location(specific): _____ , Location(general) _ , neighborhood , city_ _, state_ _(0 a 5)
3		**Record:** Repeat: car_ _ vase_ _brick_ _
5		**Calculation:** 100-7= __; 93-7=_____ ; 86-7= _____ ; 79-7= _____ ; 72-7= _ (0 a 5)
3		**Recent Memory:** Which three words did I ask you to repeat? _ (0 a 3)
9		Language: * Name two objects: pen _________watch_______(0 a 2) * Repeat the expression: "neither here, nor there, nor there" (0 a 1)

		* Three-step command: take this sheet of paper in your right hand, fold it in half and place it on the floor ______________________ (0 a 3) * Read to perform: Close your eyes ___ (0 a 1) * Write a complete sentence ________(0 a 1) Copy the diagram: ______ (0 a 1)
30		Note

Table 03. Source: BERTOLLUCI, BRUCKI AND CAMPACCI (1994).

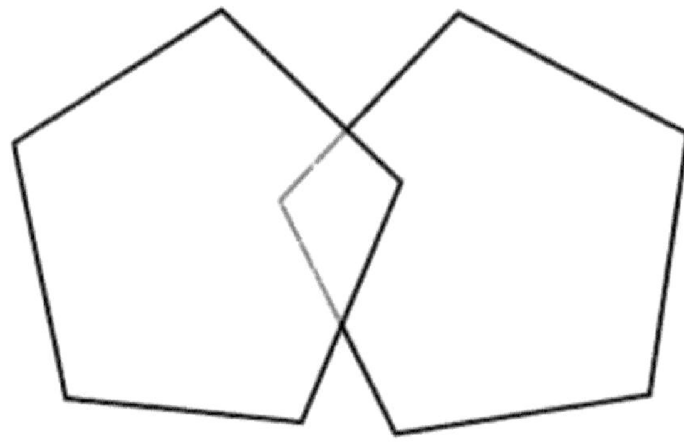

ANNEX 02 - IPAQ

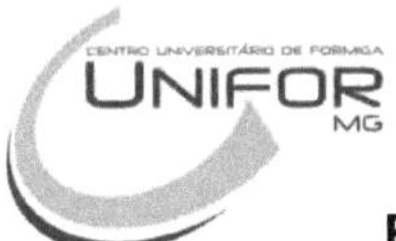

FORMIGA UNIVERSITY CENTER

Decree published on 05/08/2004

Sponsor: Fundaçâo Educacional Comunitària Formiguense - FUOM

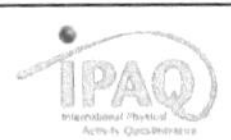

INTERNATIONAL PHYSICAL ACTIVITY QUESTIONNAIRE

Short version

Name:____

Date: _____ / ______ / _____ **Age :** ______ **Sex: F ( ) M ( )**

We are interested in finding out what kind of physical activity people do as part of their daily lives. This project is part of a larger study being carried out in different countries around the world. Your answers will help us understand how active we are compared to people in other countries. The questions relate to the amount of time you spent doing physical activity in the **LAST** week. The questions include activities you do at work, to get from one place to another, for leisure, for sport, for exercise or as part of your activities at home or in the garden. Your answers are VERY important. Please answer each question even if you think you are not active. Thank you for your participation!

To answer the questions, remember that:
> **VIGOROUS** physical activities are those that require great physical effort and make you breathe MUCH harder than normal
> **MODERATE** physical activities are those that require some physical effort and make you breathe A LITTLE harder than normal.

To answer the questions, think only about the activities you do **for at least 10 minutes** at a time.

1a On how many days in the last week did you **WALK** for at least 10 minutes continuously at home or at work, as a form of transport to get from one place to another, for leisure, pleasure or as a form of exercise?

days ____ per **WEEK** ( ) None

1b On days when you walked for at least 10 minutes continuously, how much time in total did you spend walking **each day**?

hours: _____ Minutes: ____

2a) On how many days in the last week did you do **MODERATE** activities for at least 10 minutes continuously, such as light cycling, swimming, dancing, light aerobics, playing recreational volleyball, carrying light weights, doing household chores in the house, yard or garden such as sweeping, vacuuming, tending the garden, or any activity that increased **moderately**.

your breathing or heartbeat **(PLEASE DO NOT INCLUDE WALKING)**

days ____ per **WEEK** ( ) None

2b. On the days when you did these moderate activities for at least 10 minutes continuously, how much time in total did you spend doing these activities **per day**?

hours: _____ Minutes: ____

3a On how many days in the last week did you do **VIGOROUS** activities for at least 10 continuous minutes, such as running, aerobics, playing soccer, cycling fast on a bike, playing basketball, doing heavy housework around the house, yard or garden digging, carrying heavy weights or any activity that increased your breathing or heart rate a LOT.

days ____ per **WEEK** ( ) None

3b On the days when you did these vigorous activities for at least 10 minutes continuously, how much time in total did you spend doing these activities **per day**?

hours: _____ Minutes: ____

These last questions are about the time you spend sitting every day, at work, at school or college, at home and during your free time. This includes sitting while studying, sitting while resting, doing homework, visiting a friend, reading, sitting or lying down watching TV. Do not include time spent sitting during transportation by bus, train, metro or car.

4a. How much time do you spend sitting down on a **weekday**?

hours _____ minutes

4b. How much time in total do you spend sitting down on a **weekend day**?

hours _____ minutes

Source: PARDINI, et al. (2001)

ANNEX 03 - Predicted values for muscle strength according to BLACK; HYATT (1969)

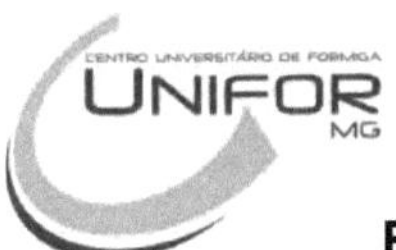

FORMIGA UNIVERSITY CENTER

Decree published on 05/08/2004

Sponsor: Fundaçâo Educacional Comunitària Formiguense - FUOM

Predicted Values for Muscle Strength
Pimâx Men = 143 - (0.55 x Age) Women = 104 - (0.51 x Age)
Pemâx Men = 268 - (1.03 x Age) Women = 170 - (0.53 x Age)

Table 04. Source: BLACK; HYATT (1969).

ANNEX 04 - Consubstantiated Opinion of the UNIFOR-MG Research Ethics Committee

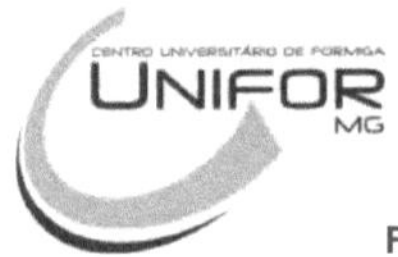

FORMICA UNIVERSITY CENTER

ACCREDITATION Decree Published on 05/08/2004

RECREDENTIALIZATION: Decree Published on 15/12/2006

Sponsor: Fundação Educacional Comunitária Formiguense - FUOM

CONSUBSTANTIATED **PÀRËCER**

OpinionN ⁰ 01/2012

Principal Investigator: Ana Paula de Lourdes Pfister

Executive team: Ligia Pelosi Mendonça

Type of Research: Capstone - Physiotherapy

CEPH/UNIFOR registration: 11/11/2011 Process N ⁰ 101/2011

Institution where it will be developed: Dental Clinic Dr. Arthur Lopes Mendonça/ Dental Clinic Dr. Vânia Regina da Costa Pelosi

Group: III

Status: APPROVED

The Ethics Committee for Research Involving Humans of the Centro Universitario de Formiga has analyzed process N.⁰ 101/2011, concerning the research project: "Evaluation of respiratory muscle strength and peak expiratory flow in individuals with Obstructive Sleep Apnea Syndrome (OSAS) and the relationship with the use of benzodiazepines" with Ana Paula de Lourdes Pfister, as the researcher in charge, whose objective is "To evaluate respiratory muscle strength and airflow obstruction in individuals with Obstructive Sleep Apnea (OSAS), as well as their relationship with benzodiazepines".

Therefore, based on the social and scientific importance of the project, its applicability and compliance with ethical requirements, we are in favor of the project being carried out and classify it as APPROVED, as it meets the fundamental requirements of Resolution 196/96 and its Complementary Resolutions of the National Health Council/MS.

The researcher is asked to send CEPH-UNIFOR partial reports whenever there are any changes to the project, as well as the final report saved on CD-ROM.

Formiga, February 10, 2012.

Formiga, 10 de fevereiro de 2012

Ivani Pose Martins
Presidenta do CEPH/UNIFOR

AV. DR. ARNALDO DE SENNA, 328 - ÁGUA VERMELHA - CEP: 35570-000 - FORMIGA -MG- FONE: (37) 3329-1438

HTTP7/WWW UNIFORMG EDU BR - E-MAIL: COMITEDEETICA@UNIFORMG.EDU.BR

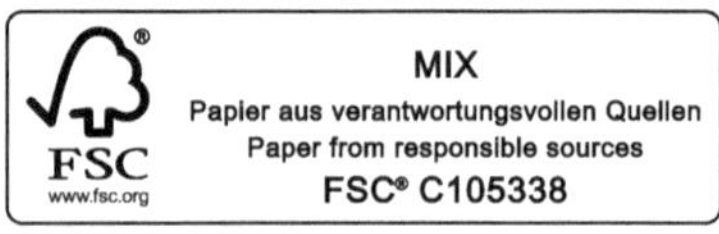

Printed by Books on Demand GmbH, Norderstedt / Germany